Nature Will Heal Acne.

In nature's arms, we find our cure,
Her gentle touch, our skin's allure.
With earth's own gifts, we softly tend,
To nurture, heal, our skin's best friend

Disclaimer

This ebook is intended for educational and promotional purposes only. This ebook was written with precision and comprehensiveness in mind. However, typographical and grammatical errors may exist. Additionally, the data in this ebook is only current as of the date it was written.

The target audience for this ebook is students. Neither the author nor the publisher guarantees the accuracy or completeness of any of the information presented in this ebook. Neither the author nor the publisher will be held liable for any direct or indirect damages that might be incurred as a result of using this ebook.

Acne is a skin disorder that manifests itself in the hair follicles and is caused by an overproduction of oil. Puberty triggers the activation of these glands because of the simultaneous release of male and female hormones. Acne is common during this time due to fluctuating hormone levels. Acne develops when oil from the skin's oil glands at the base of hair follicles becomes trapped.Although acne has no serious health risks, it can be distressing and socially uncomfortable, especially for teenagers. Between the ages of 11 and 30, acne affects an estimated 75% of the population. In addition to the face, other common locations for acne breakouts are the back, chest, shoulders, and neck.

Recent studies suggest a genetic component to acne vulnerability. Acne in the mother is a strong indicator that the child will also suffer from the condition. Androgen and lithium-containing medicines have the potential to exacerbate acne. Those who are prone to acne should avoid using oil-based cosmetics, since they might exacerbate the condition. Acne, either new or old, can appear or return during pregnancy because of hormonal shifts.

Acne Subtypes

- Whiteheads are a subcutaneous kind of acne that rarely shows on the surface of the skin.

- Visible blackheads are not the result of dirt buildup, and neither will they disappear no matter how often you wash your face.

- Papules, which are superficial pink pimples, can be seen on the skin's surface.

Red pimples with pus on top of the skin are called pustules.

- Nobules are large, firm, painful pimples. They form deep within the dermis.

What seems like a minor annoyance to most people might be a major problem for others. Pus-filled cysts are quite uncomfortable.

When you go to the movies, you see stunning actors with flawless complexions. Maybe you've even felt a twinge of envy towards them. However, it's possible that their skin isn't actually as "perfect" as you may assume. Acne is a problem that many prominent people, including Jessica Simpson, Kelly Clarkson, and Katy Perry, have openly discussed. They may have had "glowing" skin onstage thanks to cosmetics, but they all suffered from the same skin care issue that millions of people around the world do: acne.

Acne is a common side effect of puberty. Acne is often a result of hormonal imbalances and the resulting hormonal fury. At that age, even a single zit might feel like the end of the world. Acne is a common skin condition, but for some people it's simply a minor issue that clears up fast. However, for some people it is a nightmare. Nothing they try seems to stop the acne from covering their face. Even in maturity, it continues to plague certain people. These people usually have it so severe that they are permanently damaged by it. Having acne isn't just inconvenient; it can also be humiliating. Particularly during the while you're in your teens and self-respect is crucial. It's a fact that youngsters can be harsh, and that those with severe acne are sometimes the subject of their bullying. They are the target of verbal abuse and/or mockery. This causes them a great deal of anxiety, which in turn exacerbates their acne. There may be a spiralling effect.

What can you do if you're one of the unfortunate persons that suffers from acne? Commercials abound encouraging you to get rid of acne by using the advertised product or cleaner. Trying to make a purchase decision can be a frustrating experience. It can cost hundreds of dollars for some folks to find the correct product. As a result, they waste a lot of money on useless things.

Salicylic acid can be used to unclog pores and benzoyl peroxide can be found in many over-the-counter lotions and gels for treating acne.

Acne-fighting prescriptions can take the form of either oral antibiotics or topical antimicrobials. Some oral contraceptives for women can help reduce oil production by calming the glands that produce sebum.

If these don't help, your doctor may recommend more invasive procedures. Chemical peels are commonly used to exfoliate dead skin and unclog pores.

If you decide to take this path, it's important to pick a dermatologist with care. Some of them have never dealt with acne before. Verify their credentials by requesting before-and-after pictures of people who underwent the same procedure you're considering. They ought to be able to provide you with "before" and "after" pictures.

If you've never dealt with acne, you have no idea how much money may go into treating it. Among the potential expenses associated with medical approaches to acne skin treatment are the following:

- Nonprescription, everyday use of a cleanser, toner, and medicated lotion might set you back $30 to $60 a month

- Treatment can cost anywhere from $50 to $200 per month with a medical visit if it is severe and antibiotics, topical creams, ointments, or hormone therapy are prescribed.

Facials and chemical peels are two methods that some people use to combat acne. One session of these treatments can cost $75 to $200, and you may need multiple sessions per month.

- Scarring from acne occurs in some persons. Patients with acne scars may opt for more extensive treatments in hopes of erasing or minimising their appearance. Scarring treatments, whether they be microdermabrasion or dermabrasion, can cost up to $2,000 if multiple sessions are required.

Acne can be treated successfully with medication, but maintenance care is necessary to prevent further breakouts. Cosmetic medical procedures are sometimes not covered by health insurance. New patients are often given special offers for skin resurfacing procedures by their doctors. If you require 6 of something, they might have bundle deals.

- Different therapies. Generic versions of brand-name meds are also widely available. Up to a 50% savings is possible with these.

The costs associated with several common medical procedures are as follows:

The price of a 45-gram tube of tretinoin ranges from $35 to $50, depending on the potency.

- Adapalene, a generic with varying concentrations. It's a hefty sum. A 45-gram tube can set you back around $160.

Epiduo combines adapalene and benzoyl peroxide under a single brand name. Up to $250 can be spent on a 45-gram container of this gel. Because benzoyl peroxide can be purchased so cheaply on its own, you may decide that purchasing the antibiotic and benzoyl peroxide combo is not worth the extra money.

The microsphere preparation of trentinoin found in Retin-A Micro, which may be less irritating, is another option. The price of a 45 gramme tube can range from $260 to $320. In comparison, the cost of living in the United States is a lot cheaper in other countries

.

• Tazorac is effective for both acne and psoriasis. It gets the job done, but it also has a reputation for being annoying. The price range for just 30 grammes of this gel is $200-$250.

• Benzaclin, which consists of 1% clindamycin and 5% benzoyl peroxide, is a bit cheaper. A 25-gram tube will run you between $75 and $95.

• Duac - A more expensive brand-name alternative to Benzaclin gel. Over $200 can be spent on 45 grammes.

The cost of 30 grammes of Ziana ranges from $225 to $250. The combined cost of clindamycin and tretinoin, two generics, can be anywhere from $50 to $100.

• Doxycycline is a prescription antibiotic that is taken twice day in doses of 50 mg to 100 mg. It's generic, so a month's supply will only set you back about $4.

• Acne can be treated with Oracea, a 40 mg pill. It accomplishes its purpose but at a high cost. A month's supply might cost as much as $400.

• Taken twice daily, minocycline is less likely to cause a sunburn-inducing rash than doxycycline. A month's supply of the drug in dosages ranging from 50 mg to 100 mg can be purchased for as little as $12 to $30.

• Solodyn–This is an extended-release type of minocycline. While it is more practical than daily dosage, the cost can range from $560 to $1,000 per month.

It's clear that people with acne have a high propensity to spend money. It's frequently wasted because the lotions and medicines are ineffective. Despite your best efforts, your skin condition persists despite your best efforts to clear it up.

Would you attempt a method to get rid of acne if you knew it wouldn't cost you anything? This might turn out to be the situation for you. Perhaps there is already something in your kitchen or bathroom that will serve the purpose.

Frustration builds when you realise you can't stop the changes appearing on your face. Many people have bad acne breakouts after using every over-the-counter remedy and every medicine their doctor prescribes. However, sometimes neither dermatologists nor drugs are the answer. Instead, we might look to nature for the solution. Acne can be treated well using natural therapies. Natural remedies are safer for your skin and can be as effective as their high-priced counterparts.

50 WAYS TO TREAT ACNE USING NATURAL REMEDIES

If you're one of those who suffer from severe acne, you're probably willing to try just about anything. If you've tried and tried to clear your face of acne and you've used every cleanser or acne cream you can think of and you are still plagued with acne, you should know that there are many natural ways to help you clear up your acne and often get rid of it permanently. You don't have to waste money, and most of these things you already have around your house. If you think this sounds too good to be true, trust me, it isn't.

You can have clearer skin in a short period of time for far less money than you'd spend buying medical creams and pills. Often, you don't have to use anything. You just have to adjust a few things that you do in your daily routine to help clear up your acne. Wouldn't that be awesome? Natural remedies have worked for others, and these remedies can work for you too. Try several of these methods until you find the combination of natural products that work for you.

Here are 50 tips you can use that will naturally help you clear up that dreaded acne and reclaim healthy, clear skin:

1. Baking Soda–When you think baking soda, you probably think of keeping your refrigerator fresh. Baking soda, in fact, does much more. For acne, mix baking soda and water in equal parts. Use them to make a paste you can apply to your face. Don't put it all over your face. You'll only want to put it on each individual acne spot. It's usually easier to use a Q-Tip and dab it on. Leave it on your face until it dries. This usually takes around 10

minutes. Wash it off in water that is very cold. This helps close pores. Generally, doing this twice each day can give results.

2. Lemon Juice–Lemons have citric acid which fights bacteria that cause acne. It's easy to use as an acne treatment. Simply cut a lemon in half. Then rub the open side of the lemon gently on your face. You will feel it stinging, which mean it is working. Leave it on for about 10 minutes. Be sure to wash the lemon juice off. When you use lemon juice for your acne, you probably should use sunscreen if you're going outdoors. The citric acid can sometimes bleach the skin. This can make your skin more sensitive and makes it a higher risk for sun damage.

3. Potatoes–Slice a small, raw potato in half. Rub it on the acne. You want to rub it only on the affected areas, not your entire face. Potatoes not only have a healing effect, but are also an anti-inflammatory. This will help with that embarrassing and irritating swelling and redness acne can have on your face.When you're finished, wash the potato residue off of your face gently.

4. Toothpaste–This works well for pimples. If you have one or two that you want to get rid of quickly, simply apply toothpaste to it. Toothpaste contains silica which dries out and reduces the size of the pimple overnight if you leave it on. Toothpaste that has silica but not sodium lauryl sulfate works best. Most big name- brand toothpastes have sodium lauryl sulfate, so stick with the simple, natural ones when you use it to treat your acne.

5. Ice–Ice has been used for years to treat inflammation in the body. That's why when there's swelling from any kind of an injury, ice is applied to the affected area. For acne, ice is used because it closes pores as well as helps reduce the inflammation of acne. If you have big pores, you can take ice cubes and rub them gently over the problem spots. Ice or even cold packs, work to constrict blood vessels beneath the skin. This causes irritation and/or inflammation to be less noticeable.

6. Tea Tree Oil–It is a well-known anti-fungal and antibacterial remedy. It's herbal, so it's great for mild-moderate acne. In tests, it has been just as effective as benzoyl peroxide for acne. The benzoyl peroxide may work more quickly, but teal tree oil will have fewer side effects and treat your acne naturally.

7. Aspirin–You'll want to crush the aspirin and form a paste. Then use a Q-Tip or your finger to apply the paste on each pimple and let it dry. Aspirin contains salicylic acid. They use this in most acne treatments, because it will destroy bacteria which cause acne. It dries out pimples while it fights bacteria. Leave the mixture on your face for 10-15 minutes and wash off gently.

8. Alum–You can check the spice aisle in your local grocery store and look for Potassium alum. It is also used in natural deodorants and styptic to help reduce bleeding after a cut because it's a natural antiseptic and astringent that shrinks skin tissue. It works better in block form than power.

Just wipe it over your acne gently to avoid irritating pimples.

9. Reduce refined carbohydrates from your diet –Things like bread, pasta, etc. can cause your acne to worsen. You should also try to cut back on sugar. You may want to use a little natural sugar, but eating a lot of sweets will negatively affect your acne. When you're looking for something to munch on, instead of candy bars, go for things that are healthier, such as fruits and vegetables.

10. Fermented foods–Foods such as sauerkraut, kefir, natural yogurt or goat cheese contain pro-biotic and enzymes which help reduce acne. Adding these to your diet can be beneficial when you're struggling with acne breakouts.

11. Stop using products on your face such as cleansers, makeup, and face cream–If you feel you need these things, you should look until you find natural products. Often these products aren't

made to work together. If you're trying natural ways to cure your acne, then don't counteract the effect with other chemical products.

12. Vegetables–You've been told all your life it's important to eat your vegetables. If you have acne problems, you should definitely add more vegetables to your daily diet. They're healthy, and they clean toxins from your blood that can cause acne.

13. Water–Drinking water also helps cleanse the body. You should try to get about half your body weight in ounces of water daily. As the water cleanses your body, it will help cleanse the pores of the skin and keep them from clogging. If you drink more water instead of soft drinks, you'll probably not only see a difference in your acne, but your health in general.

14. Be active–Moving around helps your lymphatic system. Try doing things such as running, jumping rope, or even jumping on a trampoline. Join a gym and workout. Join a sports

team in school or at your local YMCA. Whatever activity you enjoy that gets you moving. Often when one suffers from acne they stay home and seem to become a young couch potato. They don't want to go anywhere or do anything where others will see their acne. Forget about that. Don't worry about others, worry about yourself. You need to move, so get out and do it. Run laps around your yard if necessary, but move!

15. Vitamin A–Taking a multivitamin is good whether or not you have acne, but it is proven that Vitamin A does help reduce acne. You should try to get a vitamin that has a good supply of Vitamin A, because it helps regenerate skin. It can reduce wrinkles and help get rid of blemishes.

16. Keep your face clean–You can use simple soap and wash your face at least twice a day. If your skin tends to be oily, you should rinse it several times throughout the day. Use lukewarm water to help remove oil that leads to breakouts. You should use mild soap and a soft washcloth or

soft sponge. Strong soaps and rough material will irritate acne. Just a little soap is enough. Make sure you rinse it thoroughly. After washing splash your face with cool water to close your pores. When you're finished, pat your face dry–don't rub it.

17. Sleep well–The more you sleep, the less stressed you'll be. Every hour you lose of sleep causes you around 15% more stress. This can cause the hormones to go crazy causing acne. Instead of staying up late watching TV, or cramming for that test you forgot to study for, you should go to bed at a decent hour.

18. No popping or picking–If you're doing everything you can using natural remedies to treat your acne, it can be useless if you pop or pick at your acne. You may want to, but it won't be good for you in the long run. Acne is bacteria and when you pop it, you allow it to spread to more pores. In effect, you're spreading bacteria to the pores you just cleaned. That's not a good idea. Popping and picking acne also causes

inflammation which can cause the acne to appear worse, and cause you to have scars.

19. Avoid glycemic foods–Foods with high glycemic content are not good for acne. This includes: soft drinks, white bread, rice, potatoes, beer, cake, and commercial cereals to name a few. Making a few changes in your diet, like substituting a baked sweet potato for your usual loaded baked potato, eating whole wheat cereals, or buying pasta enriched with soy protein can help reduce your glycemic intake.

20. Baby powder–Baby powder has long been used to absorb moisture. Lightly rub your face with baby powder before you go to bed and when you get up in the morning. The baby powder will keep your face dry and oil-free and will help dry up blemishes.

21. Honey–Use a honey mask on your face a few times a week. Honey is an antibacterial, and can disinfect and help heal blemishes. It is gentle

enough for even the most sensitive skin. You use the honey like you would any commercial facial mask. Just rub the honey on your entire face. Let it sit until it's totally dry, and then peel it off.

22. Keep your hair away–Your hair contains oil and can help lead to breakouts. Wash your hair everyday and after every workout. If your hair is long or you have bangs, be sure to pull your hair away from your face. Cleaning your face and then allowing your hair to be on it can reduce the effect of your cleansing. Many people use their hair to hide their acne. They keep their hair over as much of their face as possible. You're not the first person to have severe acne, and you won't be the last. Pull your hair back and don't worry who sees it. You may be self conscious at first, but when your acne begins to clear, you'll be glad you did it.

23. Eat carrots–Carrots have beta-carotene or Vitamin A–They help strengthen your protective tissue and prevent acne. It is also a good antioxidant which can help rid your body of

toxins. Carrots are great for a snack and are much better to nibble on while you do your homework than chips or cookies.

24. Clean pillowcases–Your face lays on your pillow daily. The pillowcase can absorb oil from your skin. If your wash your face before you go to bed and lay your head on a dirty pillowcase, you're reapplying the dirt and oil. This renders your cleansing useless. You should wash your pillowcase at least every other day. This way, you will get the most from your natural treatments.

25. Eat foods with Zinc–Look for foods that are high in Zinc. It is an antibacterial agent necessary in your skin's oil-producing. Not getting enough Zinc can actually cause breakouts. There are many foods high in Zinc such as: oysters, wheat germ, veal liver, roast beef, roasted pumpkin and squash, dark chocolate, lamb, peanuts, and crab. Adding some of these to your diet can help fight your acne.

26. Avoid smoking–You know smoking is bad for you. It damages many parts of your body and causes multiple health problems.

For acne, smoking can clog pores and increase breakouts.

27. No excessive sunbathing–Some sun is good for you, but if you're going to be in the sun for some time, be sure to wear SPF. You're probably using a lot of products either commercial or natural on your face. Many of these react to extreme sunlight. Using SPF will help take care of your skin.

28. Rose water glycerine–Rose water glycerine makes a good facial rinse. After cleaning your face, using rose water glycerine as a rinse can help remove residue and other pollutants. It leaves your face cleaner than just with soap and water.

29. Don't touch–You have no idea how many surfaces your hands touch each day. They are

constantly in contact with dirt and germs. When you touch your face, rub your eyes, etc, you just transfer all of that dirt and germs onto your face. It's a good idea to wash your hands frequently as a general rule of health. If you find it difficult not to touch your face, make sure you wash your hands often. If possible, however, avoid touching your face.

30. Don't drink alcohol–Excessive consumption of alcohol can enlarge the blood vessels that are near your skins surface.

31. Don't use multiple skincare products–You should never mix any kind of products from your pharmacy, including skincare products. Some don't work well with others. Others will have the same ingredients. This means you're getting too much of it and can help increase the problem. If you find a skincare product that works, stick with it and get rid of the others. Once you find natural ways to cleanse your face and prevent acne that work, just do away with the store-bought ones.

32. Grapeseed oil–Add a teaspoon of grapeseed oil to whichever toner you use. It can help your skin cells damaged by acne repair themselves.

33. Apple cider vinegar/rubbing alcohol/lemon juice toner–Don't mix them together, but individually, these work well. These both kill dead skin cells and clean out pores because they are highly acidic. You do have to be careful when you use them. If your skin starts to dry out, you can use the one you choose less often or use water to dilute it a bit.

34. Brown sugar–Your pores will open up after a shower since your skin is wet. Scrub the affected areas with brown sugar to reduce acne. In addition to reducing acne, it also aids in maintaining smooth skin. Scrubbing your skin every day is not recommended. At least twice a suffice for a month.

35. Egg whites, a natural oil-controlling ingredient. Simply remove the whites from one or two eggs. If the whites are inconsistent, beat

them until they are. Apply the whites all over your face and let them sit there for around fifteen to twenty minutes before washing. It will leave your face less oily, which is a huge plus when it comes to clearing up acne.

36. Egg yolks–the yolks aid in preventing blocked pores. Retinoids, a form of Vitamin A, are present in it. Numerous cosmetics contain this Retin-A. Assume the worst and assume the best. Keep them on your face for 15 to 20 minutes until they have hardened, and then remove them and wash your face. If you do this once a week, you won't have to worry about your pores getting clogged up.

37. Garlic–Although its efficacy hasn't been scientifically confirmed, anecdotal evidence suggests it may help. Just take two garlic cloves, peel them, and mash them up. Apply the extracted juice to your face. Turn it on and let it run for 5-10 minutes. You're free to use it as much as you like, but keep it off for too long at a time.

38. Mint, or mint, is a natural skin soother. They have the pain reliever menthol in them. They reduce the redness that often accompanies acne. Use the extract from mint leaves mint oil, or mint leaves. Apply it for ten to fifteen minutes, then wash your face thoroughly. Since it's an anti-inflammatory, you can use it as much as you like without worrying about damaging your skin.

39. Combine one teaspoon of cinnamon with one teaspoon of honey. Apply and leave on your face for 15 minutes. Use warm water and pat dry afterward. Antiviral, antifungal, and antibacterial characteristics are just a few of the benefits associated with cinnamon. Honey's antibacterial properties allow it to promote speedy recovery and comfort. It can also absorb moisture thanks to its hygroscopic nature.

40. Making your own plain yoghurt at home is preferable to buying it from the store if you know how. In any case, plain yoghurt is the way to go. Get rid of dull skin with a yoghurt face pack and

20 minutes of rest. Get some warm water and wash it off. It's cleansing, refreshing, and calming, all in one.

41. Homemade facial oil for acne–Combining several natural oils yields an effective facial oil that also helps to hydrate the skin. About a single ounce of jojoba oil will do the trick. Oils of carrot seed, lavender, and geranium, three drops each. Blend the ingredients together, then dab a small quantity of the oil on your face using your fingertips.

42. Clove oil–You shouldn't use pure clove oil to your face, as it will cause irritation. Discover a top-notch clove oil mixture. It's helpful for the extremely painful cystic acne. It's an overnight topical therapy that helps clear up acne.

43. Loosen your sporting gear; headbands and helmets, in particular, can exacerbate acne around the hairline and should be avoided. They can be caused by the rubbing of a helmet's chin

strap against the user's skin. In order to allow your skin to breathe, you should loosen or remove these items when you're not using them for your sport.

44. Take a shower after exercising of any kind; whether you hit the gym, the field, the court, the court or the court, your body will sweat. When this occurs, it aids in the exfoliation of dead skin. That's great, as exercise is essential for clearing up acne, but all that sweating will leave you covered in salt. The salt will clog your pores if you don't wash it off.

45. Master the art of stress management; the pressures of modern life, especially for teenagers, can be overwhelming. Acne can be a source of stress at times. This will simply make your acne worse. Hormones that are released into the bloodstream in response to stress. It has a profound effect on the skin and causes oil production to rise. Seek it out exercise that puts you at ease and lowers your stress levels. Getting outside and walking around can do wonders for

clearing your mind. Making sure your assignments aren't last-minute scrambles and giving yourself plenty of time to study for tests are also helpful strategies. Everything that puts you under stress or strain must be addressed and controlled well.

46. Indian cuisine typically makes use of the spice turmeric. Adding it to eggs or stir-fry is a great way to add flavour while cooking at home. It can reduce swelling and pain and kill germs. Acne redness and irritation may be alleviated.

47. Use device-safe antibacterial wipes to clean your mobile phone, sunglasses, or conventional glasses whenever they come into contact with your face. In the same way that you wouldn't want to put your unclean hands on your face, you also shouldn't put your dirty equipment near your face. You know you don't want to if you've already made up your mind.

48. Reduce your dairy consumption; research has shown that an increase in oil production from the oil glands is negative for acne. Some products can be swapped out for others, including substitute nondairy milk (such as soy or coconut milk) for cow's milk to cut down on dairy consumption and oil use.

49. Banana peels - Try rubbing a tiny piece of banana peel on the pimple for a few minutes. It needs to be rubbed until the pulp inside the peel turns brown. The skin absorbs the peel's vitamins and nutrients when the peel's particles dry on it. Wash it off with warm water after about 30 minutes of application. Repeat thrice daily. The peel particles can be left on the face overnight before being washed off in the morning.

50. Papaya – You'll find papaya extract in many advertising cosmetics today. However, you need not spend a lot of money on Papaya products in order to reap their benefits. Raw papaya is considerably more effective, and it can be used to treat acne naturally. It aids in the elimination of excess lipids and dead skin cells. The papain enzyme that papayas contain is anti-

inflammatory as well. It's simple to operate. Use water to wash your face, then pat it dry. You should thoroughly crush the papaya's flesh. The consistency should be such that it may be spread easily throughout the skin. Apply it where it hurts. For best results, let it sit on your skin for around 20 minutes before rinsing. Wash with tepid water and blot dry. Finding a natural moisturiser that works with your skin type is essential if your skin dries up after cleansing.